Ketogenic Diet for Beginners and the Keto Lifestyle Plan

All You Need to Know to Control Weight

and Live A Healthy Life

DAVID LIBERATO

Dedication

To my wife and my lovely daughter….

Table of Contents

Introduction

Congratulations on downloading your copy of the *Ketogenic Diet for Beginners and Keto Lifestyle Plan: All You Need to Know to Control Weight and to Live A Healthy Life.* I am so excited that you have chosen to take a new path using the Ketogenic diet plan. The plan is recognized by several names including the low-carb diet, Ketogenic low-carbohydrate diet & high-fat (LCHF) diet plan, and the Keto diet.

Your liver produces ketones which are used as energy to provide sufficient levels of protein. The process of ketosis is natural and happens every day – no matter the total of carbs consumed. Before you begin the journey to ketosis; here is a bit of insight on how the diet plan was discovered:

During the course of history as early as the 20th century, fasting was theorized by Bernarr Macfadden as a means for restoring your health. One of his students introduced a treatment for epilepsy using the same plan. In 1912, it was reported by the *New York Medical Journal* that the fast is a successful method to treat epileptic patients, followed by a starch- and sugar-free diet.

In 1921, Rollin Woodyatt noted the ketone bodies (three water-soluble compounds, β-hydroxybutyrate, acetone, and acetoacetate) were produced by the liver as a result of a diet low in carbohydrates and rich in fat.

Also, in 1921, Dr. Russell Wilder worked for the Mayo Clinic and became well-known when he formulated the keto plan, which was then used as part of the epilepsy therapy treatment plan at that time. He had a huge interest in the plan because he also suffered from epilepsy. The plan became known for its other effects which helped in weight loss, and many other ailments.

The ketosis dieting technique was set aside in the 1940s because "improved" methods were discovered for the treatment of epilepsy. However, during that time - approximately 30% of the cases using these alternate plans had failed. Therefore, the original ketogenic plan was reintroduced to the patients. As of 2016, Wilder is still functioning successfully without seizure episodes.

As a direct result of Dr. Wilder's discovery, innovation began at the Mayo Clinic. Another physician standardized the diet plan using the following calculation:

- 10-15 carbs daily

- 1 gram of protein per kilogram of bodyweight
- The remainder of the count will remain with fat

As time passed, the plan had a few changes to make it functional as it is today.

The Charlie Foundation was founded by the family of Charlie Abraham in 1994 after his recovery from daily seizures, and other health issues. Charlie — as a youngster — was placed on the diet and continued to use it for five years. As of 2016, he is still functioning successfully without seizure episodes and is furthering his education as a college student.

The Charlie Foundation appointed a panel of dietitians and neurologists to form an agreement in the form of a statement in 2006. It was written as an approval of the diet and stated under which cases its use would be considered. It is noted that the plan is especially recommended for children.

Chapter 1:

The Ketogenic Diet & Its Benefits

You may find the keto plan a bit challenging at first because it takes a lot of willpower to count those carbs. However, that is one huge benefit while you are on the ketogenic plan because the meals taste delicious.

Before You Get Started

Clear the temptations and prepare your kitchen with essential food items to make your diet successful. Prepare for the diet using the following tips:

Remove Temptations: Remove the candy, rice, pasta, bread, and sugary sodas you have supplied in your kitchen. If you live alone, this is an easy task. It is a bit more challenging if you have a family. The keto diet will also be excellent for them if you're using the recipes included in this book.

Market Time: When you go to the supermarket, take your new skills, a grocery list, and be sure to take plenty of time to read the labels.

Calculate All Carbs: Products consumed today have the nutritional labels on the package. Take a bit of extra time when you plan a shopping adventure. It is essential to check the panels on every item to keep the ketosis in line. It might be a complicated process at first, but it is worth the effort.

Prepare a Journal of all Food Eaten: If you cheat on the intake of carbs, your additional carbohydrate points must be counted in your daily totals. It will be a reminder of your indulgence, but it will help keep you in line. It is your health and well-being that you are improving.

Purchase a Food Scale: Keeping accurate records is essential to know how many carbs, fats, and proteins you are consuming. Guesswork can be costly such as a 6-ounce steak could very well be an 8-ounce piece of meat. You have to be precise to keep your body in the right mode. These are some of the options you should consider when you buy a new food scale:

- Removable Plate: For health reasons, a removable plate will allow you to keep the germs at 'bay' for easy cleaning.

- Automatic Shut-off: Search for a scale that doesn't have an auto shut-off button. Nothing is more frustrating than to be adding your meal totals, and it shuts off!

- Have a Conversion Button: Many of the websites and recipe apps use different units of measure. It is beneficial to have one that can convert the ounces to grams for easy measuring of your food items.

- Tare Function: A tare feature will allow you to set the scale back to zero when you place plates, bowls, or other items on the scale.

Weigh the Now and Later: It is always tempting to test your loyalty to the diet and exercise plan you have chosen. You will need to learn how to pass by that sugary sundae you are craving. You'll be happier in the long-term by continuing on the right path to weight loss and not cheating with the loaded calories.

Vital Roles of Protein & Calories

Protein & Its Importance

Protein is a must for your dieting plan for these reasons:

Muscle Repair and Growth: Protein should be increased on days you are more active. It's essential to have a plan and understand the balance of carbs, proteins, and fats. The balance is the goal you are attempting to achieve, and it's found in a focused plan such as the keto diet.

Protein Saves Your Calories: Protein slows down your digestion process making you feel more satisfied with the foods you consume. During the first segment of your diet plan, it's imperative that you feel full, so there is no temptation to cheat with your menu selection.

Protein is a Fat Burner: Science has proven your body can't use and burn your fat as quickly as energy sources produce - unless you have help from either carbs or protein. The balance of protein must be maintained to preserve your calorie-burning lean muscles.

Carbohydrates

Your body exchanges 100% of the carbs your intake and turns it into glucose which gives your body an energy boost. About 50%-60% of your intake of calories is produced by those carbs which are stored in your liver as glycogen and is released as your body needs it.

Glucose is essential for the creation of adenosine triphosphate (ATP) which is an energy molecule. The fuel from glucose is vital for the daily maintenance and activities inside your body. After the liver has reached its maximum capacity for its limits, the excessive carbohydrates turn into fat.

The Difference Between a Low-Carb & Ketogenic Diet Plan

Don't get a low-carb diet confused with a keto diet. A low-carb diet will average 200 (+) carbs and then change to under 100 grams daily. Your long-term effect of a low-carb diet plan may differ greatly depending on the number of fats and proteins that are consumed.

How the Plan Operates

A ketogenic diet will help you reduce your calorie intake to below the volume of calories your body can expend in one day. You must retrieve the energy which is stockpiled in the fat cells to deliver energy/fuel to your muscles.

The keto diet will limit the volume of carbohydrates you consume. A substantial percentage of your fuel for the day will come from fat transformed to ketones. Once you have the protein, carbohydrates, and fat ratio monitored by the diet plan such as shown in this cookbook; you are well on the way to a successful diet strategy.

You won't eliminate fat or carbs which make it a useful and safe diet plan for fat loss. You will not be over-eating with large portions of protein. If you take the approach of eating less, without considering your diet - you will be losing essential minerals and vitamins you need daily - which can result in muscle spasms, fatigue, mental fogginess, hunger, headaches, irritability, insomnia, and emotional depression. You can also lose valuable muscle mass; not just the pounds you intended to drop.

Once you begin your lower carb keto plan, you can reduce your calorie counts, and carbohydrates; you are nurturing your body with a balanced amount of water, meat, eggs, fish, veggies, and nuts, as well as high-quality oils which allows you to lose fat without the unpleasant side effects.

Techniques Used for the Ketogenic Diet Plan

The route you choose will involve flexibility or strictness. Depending on your situation, you may not have the same goals as another person. These three categories are the possible levels for you to choose from before you begin. For now, as a beginner, you will be using the first method.

Ketogenic Plan # 1: The standard ketogenic diet (SKD) consists of moderate protein, high-fat, and is low in carbs.

Ketogenic Plan # 2: The targeted keto diet (TKD), will provide you with a technique to add carbs to the diet plan during the times when you are working out.

Ketogenic Plan # 3: The cyclical ketogenic diet (CKD) is observed with five-keto days followed by two high-carbohydrate days.

Ketogenic Plan # 4: The high-protein keto diet is comparable to the standard keto plan (SKD) in all aspects. However, it does have more protein.

Elements of Ketosis: Lipogenesis & Glycogenesis

Two elements that occur when your body doesn't need the glucose:

The Stage of Lipogenesis: If there is a sufficient supply of glycogen in your liver and muscles, any excess is converted to fat and stored.

The Stage of Glycogenesis: The excess of glucose converts to glycogen and is stored in the muscles and liver. Research indicates that only about half of your energy used daily can be saved as glycogen. When the fatty acid molecules and glycerol are released, the ketogenesis process begins and creates acetoacetate.

The acetoacetate is changed into two types of ketone units:

- *Beta-hydroxybutyrate or BHB:* Your muscles will convert the acetoacetate into BHB which will fuel your brain after you have been on the keto diet for a short time.

- *Acetone:* This is mostly excreted as waste but can also be metabolized into glucose. This is the reason individuals on a ketogenic diet will experience a distinctive smelly breath.

Your body will have no more food (as when you are sleeping). Thus - your body burns the fat to create ketones. Once the ketones break down the fats - which generate fatty acids - they will burn-off in the liver through beta-oxidation. Thus, when you no longer have a supply of glycogen or glucose, ketosis begins and will use the consumed/stored fat as energy.

Use the keto calculator via the Internet at "keto-calculator.ankerl.com." You can check your levels when you want to know what essentials your body needs during the course of your dieting plan or afterward. Just document your personal information such as height and weight into the calculator, and it will provide you with the essential math.

Benefits of the Healthy Ketogenic Lifestyle Plan

The ketogenic diet is an excellent plan and aids in the following illnesses:

For the Overweight & Obese Individuals: Many people exceed what is considered healthy figures when it comes to weight. It is imperative to use the keto diet plan to get started on the right path for weight loss.

Improved Thinking Skills: Your brain is approximately 60% fat by weight. Therefore, you might become confused as you consume high-fat foods. By increasing your fatty foods intake; you will have better chances to better your mind. It can maintain itself and work at full capacity.

Seizure Reduction for Epilepsy Patients: Reductions in seizures have occurred in children who use the ketogenic diet. The therapeutic keto diet used for epilepsy often restricts the carbs to fewer than 15 grams of carbs daily to further drive up the ketone levels. Don't try this unless you have the supervision of a medical professional.

Slowed Process of those with Alzheimer's Disease: The disease's progression can be slowed, and the symptoms reduced with the keto plan.

Cancer Patient Relief: Several types of cancer and slow tumor growths are being treated by using the keto diet technique.

Gum Disease and Tooth Decay Issues Repaired: The pH balance in your mouth is influenced by sugar intake. Your gum issues could subside after about three months on a keto diet plan.

Lower Blood Pressures: It is wise to speak with your doctor about lowering your medications while on the plan. If you begin to feel dizzy; that is one of the first signs the lack of carbs is working.

Improvement of your Cholesterol Profile: An arterial buildup is generally associated with the triglyceride and cholesterol levels, which have been proven to improve with the keto diet plan.

Pre-diabetes and Diabetes Improvements: Excess fat is removed with the keto plan, which is what is linked to pre-diabetes, type-2 diabetes, and metabolic syndrome.

Joint Pain and Stiffness is Greatly Improved: Grain-based foods are eliminated from your diet on the keto plan. It is believed the grains can be one of the biggest causes of pain or chronic illness. After all, it has been said before, "no pain –no grain."

You just aren't hungry. The fat is naturally more sustaining than just carbs. You just need to wait a little longer to become satiated after a meal. The high-carbs will force the 'full-state' to last longer.

Chapter 2:

Achieve Super Results

You may have heard you don't have to count the calories using the ketogenic diet, but it's best you do. You have to keep the balance. Have you ever heard of macros before now? First, you need to understand it is an abbreviation of the macro-nutrients including the fats, proteins, and carbohydrates. Once you have the balance, you need to do the exercise.

Balance Your Eating Habits & Exercise

Short exercises of approximately 21 minutes daily have been scientifically proven more beneficial than longer workouts. By combining the right diet with the right exercise, you can get into shape without a lot of fancy equipment.

When you are pumping away on a stationary bike or treadmill, you're building up the cortisol in your body. Cortisol is a stress hormone that usually helps burn fat. However, if you have stressful and lengthy exercises planned, your body will move into a protection mode which will cause storage of fat around your midsection. That can put you at risk for cancer, diabetes, or heart disease.

For success. It is best to use a high-intensity interval training (HIIT) method. You can work-out in short intervals during a lunch break or any part of the day you feel the need to get moving.

Understand Your Cortisol Levels and Exercise

First, you need to understand that cortisol is a hormone which is released from your adrenal gland in response to chemical signs or other stress signals. The release of cortisol in long workouts, such as jogging, and the adverse effects of the release of high doses of cortisol for weight loss are essential elements in your successful program. The hormone creates the fight-or-flight reaction as a result of the additional activity/stress during your workout.

Balance the Carbs

You are your own boss for balancing your carbohydrate intake. The following guidelines are effective about 90% of the time:

20-50 Grams of Carbs Daily: If you have diabetes, are obese, or metabolically deranged, this is the plan for you. If you are consuming less than the 50 grams daily; your body will reach a 'ketosis state' which supplies the ketone bodies. Consider some of these:

- Plenty of low-carbohydrate veggies
- Some berries with whipped cream
- Trace carbs from foods including nuts, seeds, and avocados

50-100 Grams of Carbs Daily: You'll gradually work your way through the plan by choosing these food options:

- Plenty of veggies
- Minimal intake of starchy carbs
- 2-3 pieces of fruit each day

Moderate Carb Intake: 100-150 Grams of Carbs Daily: If you are active and lean or trying to maintain weight, choose these types of food:

- Several fruits daily

- All the veggies you can eat

As you now see, it is important to experiment and categorize where you fall on the scales before you make any changes. Also, if in doubt, it's best to seek your doctor's advice before changing your eating patterns. It's possible to reduce the need for some medications.

Chapter 3:

Helpful Tips & Pitfalls to Avoid

When you fast, the hormones in your body will change. The keto plan is similar to this process. You could achieve ketosis in just a couple of days once you have used up all of your stored glycogen. It can take a month, a week, or just a few days. It all depends on which type of method you choose (previously explained). Your protein and carbohydrate intake will determine the time. Exercise also plays a vital role.

How to Know When You Are in Ketosis

Whether you have taken any tests to discover your ketosis status, your body will exhibit physical signs to prompt you. You may have a loss of appetite, increased thirst, have bad breath, or notice a stronger urine smell. These are all clues from your body. This is how it all happens:

Bad Breath Flares: You may notice a metallic or fruity taste with an odor similar to nail polish remover. This is the by-product of acetoacetic acid (acetone) which is an obvious indication of ketosis. You may also experience a drier mouth. These changes are normal as a side effect as your body processes high-fat foods.

Once you are accustomed to the ketogenic dieting techniques, the bad breath symptoms will pass. If you are socializing, try a diet soda or a non-sugary drink. Sugar-free gum is also a quick fix. Always check the nutrition labels for carbohydrate facts; you may be surprised. Diet soda and gum is not generally allowed on the keto diet because they reduce ketones. Therefore, only use it temporarily. If you are at home, just grab the toothbrush.

Thirst is Increased: Fluid retention is increased when you are consuming carbohydrates. Once the carbs are flushed away, water weight is lost. You counter-balance by increasing your water intake since you are probably dehydrated.

The ketogenic diet requires more water since as a result, you are storing carbs. If you are dehydrated; your body can use the stored carbs to restore hydration. When you're in ketosis, the carbs are removed, and your body doesn't have the water reserves. If you have tried other diets, you might have been dehydrated, but the higher carbohydrate counts stopped you from being thirsty. Thus, the keto state is a diuretic state, so drink plenty of water daily.

Ketosis and Your Sleep Patterns: After you have a good night of sleep, your body is in ketosis since you have fasted for over eight hours, you are on the way to burning ketones. If you are new to the high-fat and low-carb dieting, the optimal fat-burning state takes time. Your body has depended on bringing in carbs and glucose; it will not readily give up carbs and start to crave saturated fats.

A restless night is also a normal side effect. Vitamin supplements can sometimes remedy the problem that can be caused by a lowered insulin and serotonin level. For a quick fix; try one-half of a tablespoon of fruit spread and a square of chocolate. It sounds crazy, but it works! However, you still need to count the carbs of your medicine.

Lowered Appetite: When you reduce your carbs and proteins, you will be increasing your fat intake. The reduced appetite comes from the multitude of fibrous veggies, fats, and satiating nutrients provided in the new diet. The 'full-factor' is a huge benefit to the ketogenic plan. It will give you one less thing to worry about – being hungry.

Pungent Urine Smells: With the high acetone levels, your urine is also a strong clue to ketosis (its darkened color).

There is no reason for concern; it's just your body adjusting to the new status.

Digestive Issues: You have made a huge change in your diet overnight. It's expected you may have problems including constipation or diarrhea when you first start the keto diet. That's why you must drink plenty of water, or you could easily become constipated because of dehydration. The low-carbs contribute to the issue.

Each person is different, and it will depend on what foods you have chosen to eat to increase your fiber intake. You may experience issues because your fiber intake may be too high in comparison to your previous diet. Try reducing new foods until the transitional phase of ketosis is concluded. It should clear up with time.

You may be lacking beneficial bacteria. Try consuming fermented foods to increase your probiotics and aid digestion. You can benefit from B vitamins, omega 3 fatty acids, and beneficial enzymes as well. Eat the right veggies and add a small amount of salt to your food to help with the movements. If all else fails, try some *Milk of Magnesia.*

Other Possible Physical Side Effects

Induction Flu: The diet can make you irritable, nauseous, a bit confused, lethargic, and possibly suffer from a lingering headache. Several days into the plan should remedy these effects. If not, add one-half of a teaspoon of salt to a glass of water, and drink it to help with the side effects. You may need to do this once a day for about the first week, and it could take about 15 to 20 minutes before it helps. It will go away!

Heart Palpitations: You may begin to feel 'fluttery' as a result of dehydration or because of an insufficient intake of salt. Try to make adjustments, but if you don't feel better quickly, you should seek emergency care.

Leg Cramps: The loss of magnesium (a mineral) can be a demon and create a bit of pain with the onset of the keto diet plan changes. With the loss of the minerals during urination, you could experience attacks of cramps in your legs.

Helpful Tips

Only Eat When You're Hungry: One outstanding benefit of the keto diet plan is that you don't stay hungry. This is a common mistake when people first start a new diet, but with the ketogenic method, you can have the fats. Carbs and fats are your two major sources of energy for your body. If you are removing the carbs, they must be replaced by fats. Remove both elements, and you would starve. By consuming natural fats, you are satisfied. Enjoy eggs, fatty fish, coconut and olive oil, bacon, meat, butter, and full-fat cream.

When your body doesn't have insulin that stores the fat, you will become a fat-burning machine and start dropping those unwanted pounds. Trust your instincts and cut out one of the meals or eat several times a day but keep track of the carbs.

The Stalling and Plateaus of Weight Loss

At first, you may not notice the weight loss. There could be days or weeks where you don't notice the changes, but slow is the best method. You are altering your lifestyle and breaking old habits. You need to remain patient because there aren't any quick fixes to weight loss.

As with any new challenge, the initial phase of a long-term challenge is difficult. Once you have discovered how easy the ketogenic plan is; you will wonder how it took you so long to try it.

Check Your Medications

It's important to inform your doctor of your weight loss program. He/she may prescribe some medicines that make you gain weight. These are a few to question:

Insulin Injections: If taken in high doses, your insulin can impede weight loss. By consuming fewer carbs, you are essentially reducing the requirement of insulin. Again, ask your healthcare professional before you make any changes.

Other Possible Medications Causing Weight Gain:

- Oral contraceptives
- Anti-Depressants
- Epilepsy drugs
- Blood pressure medications

- Allergy medicines

- Antibiotics

More Sleep & Less Stress

If you are a victim of sleep deprivation, you will understand how stressful everyday life is, even before you begin a diet plan. You may believe it's too late for you, but it isn't. Your diet plan will work, but you may need to make a few other adjustments.

Chronic stress will increase your cortisol levels – the stress hormone. With that action, your hunger levels also increase. The result is that you eat more and put on the weight. It's important to find ways to remove the stress; whether it is decluttering your home or taking a vacation.

Eliminate coffee or other forms of caffeine early in the afternoon and don't consume alcohol for at least three hours before bedtime. Alcohol will also interfere with your quality of sleep which is why you wake up feeling tired after an evening of nightclubs and boozing.

If you enjoy working out for your health, be sure to do that at least four hours before time for sleeping. Make sure your room is sufficient darkness. You will wake refreshed, ready to face your tasty ketogenic breakfast.

Chapter 4:

To Eat or Not Eat

Understanding what you should or shouldn't eat is the key that keeps the ketogenic plan working as it should. This segment will provide you with the information needed to stock in your pantry and refrigerator to maintain your level of ketosis once it is achieved. The items chosen should be readily available and clearly marked (if you choose to add the items to a jar or other container).

Pantry Items

These are just a few of the most popular items you should keep on hand to complement your ketogenic diet recipes:

- Quinoa
- Coconut flour
- Stevia or Splenda
- Natural nut butter – no sugar
- Sugar-free ketchup Sugar-free gelatin
- Unsweetened cocoa powder
- Yellow mustard

- Pickles (limit sweet or bread & butter)

Nuts and Seeds

- Almonds, walnuts, and macadamias can be eaten in small amounts and are good for your carb counts.

- Flours from nuts and seeds are good substitutes for regular flour which include milled flax seed and almond flour.

Preferred Spices

You will need to become a label reader for spices because many of the pre-made products contain sugar. Sea salt is preferred over table salt since it is typically mixed with powdered dextrose. Use these items:

- Sea Salt
- Black Pepper
- Cinnamon
- Basil
- Cayenne Pepper

- Chili Powder

- Cilantro

Protein Products

The keto plan focuses on quality proteins. You can use many of these items listed as a starting point:

- *Chicken*: Thighs, breasts, drumsticks, & ground chicken

- *Fish:* Go back to nature because it is preferable to eat any foods that are caught in the wild. Include tuna (fresh & canned), trout, salmon, snapper, catfish, flounder, cod, halibut, mahi-mahi, or mackerel as part of your diet plan.

- *Shellfish:* Choose crabs, clams, lobster, oysters, scallops, squid, shrimp, or mussels.

- *Salmon*: Fresh wild caught salmon – portioned into freezer bags

- *Poultry:* Choose from duck, chicken, pheasant, or quail.

- Turkey: Breasts & ground turkey

- *Whole Eggs:* Search for a local area market for free-range options. You can scramble, fry, boil, or devil eggs up for a picnic or any occasion.

- *Peanut Butter:* Try natural peanut butter but use caution because they do contain high counts of carbohydrates and Omega-6s. Macadamia nut butter is a wise alternative.

- *Meat:* Grass-fed is preferred because it has a better fatty acid count. Choose from lamb, veal, goat, or other wild game. Cuts of beef include flank steak, sirloin, chuck roast, lean ground beef

- *Bacon and Sausage:* Avoid bacon and sausage that has extra fillers or has been cured in sugar.

- *Pork:* Pork chops, pork loins, and ham are good options. However, you also have to beware of the added sugar.

- *Venison:* This is a healthy choice.

- *Fresh Nuts:* Macadamia, sesame seeds, flax seeds, chia seeds, etc.

Vegetables

Many of the vegetables have a lot of carbohydrates. You will want to consider these for your dieting needs:

- Asparagus

- Broccoli

- Cabbage

- Cauliflower

- Onions

- Bell pepper

- Lettuce

- Parsnips

- Radishes

- Bell Peppers

- Squash

- Peas

- Spinach

- Squash

- Turnip

- Zucchini

- Tomatoes – limited

Healthy Fats

To achieve success on the ketogenic diet, you need fats. These are some of the *good* fats you will want to keep stocked:

Monounsaturated and Saturated Fats include avocado, butter, coconut oil, egg yolks, and macadamia nuts are some of the recommended categories. These products can be incorporated into your meals using dressings, sauces, or a bit of butter on your meat.

Use non-hydrogenated lards, coconut oil, ghee, or beef tallow. Less oxidation occurs in the oil because they have higher smoke points than other oils.

Other Healthy Fats:

- Olives
- Extra-virgin olive oil (EVOO)
- Sesame oil
- Flaxseed oil
- Coconut flakes

Beverages & Dairy Products

The top of the list is to drink plenty of water. You can also choose coffee or tea (non-herbal or herbal). Products such as sugar substitutes or Crystal Lite flavor packets are okay but contain carbs if you use them for a change of pace.

It is also important to maintain your health using dairy products. It is best to choose fresh/raw or organic milk products. You can also add additional protein and calcium using non-dairy products such as cashew or almond milk. Keep these in the fridge:

- Heavy cream
- Butter
- Ghee
- Sour cream
- Cream cheese
- Parmesan cheese
- Sharp cheddar cheese

The Most Popular Ketogenic Sweeteners

Each of the following suggestions will be shown as the most popular for the majority of keto diet users. Most of your ketogenic recipes are flexible on the type of sweetener used, so it is up to you. There are a few to consider:

#1 Brand: The best all-around sweetener is Pyure's Organic All-Purpose Blend with less of a bitter aftertaste versus a stevia-based product. The blend of stevia and erythritol is an excellent alternative to baking, sweetening desserts, and various cooking needs. The substitution ratio is one teaspoon of sugar for each one-third teaspoon of Pyure. Add slowly and adjust to your taste since you can always add a bit more.

If you need powdered sugar, just grind the sweetener in a NutriBullet/blender until it's very dry.

#2 Brand: Swerve Granular Sweetener is also an excellent choice as a blend. It's made from non-digestible carbs sourced from starchy root veggies and select fruits. Give it a try if you don't like the taste of stevia.

Swerve is on the market as a one-to-one substitute. Start with ¾ of a teaspoon for every one of sugar. Increase the portion to your liking. Swerve also has its own confectioners/powdered sugar for your baking needs. On the downside, it is more expensive (about twice) than other products such as the Pyure. You have to decide if it's worth the difference.

#3 *Brand:* Xylitol is on the top of the sugary list. It is excellent for sweetening your teriyaki and BBQ sauce. It tastes just like sugar! The natural occurring sugar alcohol has the Glycemic index (GI) standing of 13. If you have tried others and weren't satisfied, this might be for you.

Xylitol is also known to keep mouth bacteria in check which goes a long way to protect your dental health. The ingredient is commonly found in chewing gum. Unfortunately, if used in large amounts, it can cause diarrhea - making gum a laxative if used in large quantities.

Urgent Note: If you have a puppy in the house, be sure to use caution since it is toxic to dogs (even small amounts).

#4 *Brand:* Stevia Drops are offered by *Sweet Leaf* and offer delicious flavors including hazelnut, vanilla, English toffee, and chocolate. Enjoy making a satisfying cup of sweetened coffee and drinks. Some individuals think the drops are too bitter. At first, use only three drops to equal one teaspoon of sugar.

#5 Brand: Lakanto's Maple-Flavored Syrup is a good choice for pancake syrup since it is monk-fruit and erythritol based. You can also choose the Golden Monk Fruit Sweetener as a brown sugar choice.

The name monk-fruit came from the Buddhist monks over 1,000 years ago and is considered a cooling agent. It may not agree with your digestive system, so use it sparingly if using in baked goods.

Supplements

The ketogenic diet has many benefits, but it's possible some of the important nutrients are being overlooked in your menu planning. You may need to supplement to replace minerals including magnesium, potassium, calcium, and sodium which comes from some of the food items not used on the keto diet. These electrolytes control muscle and nerve function and many other issues. Below are just a few of the ways you can supplement your plan:

The Electrolytes: If you have a low level of electrolytes, especially potassium and sodium, you can frequently suffer from fatigue, headaches, and constipation which is commonly called keto flu. The low-carbs also cause the kidneys to dump excess water, sodium and other valuable electrolytes that much be replenished. Consider these choices:

1. *Magnesium*: One of the most evident signs of a deficiency in magnesium is muscle cramps and fatigue. A blood test is the best way to test for possible problems. Magnesium has many benefits including good nerve and muscle function, helps maintain normal heart rhythm, assists over 300 body reactions including maintaining adequate testosterone levels and working with calcium to keep your bones healthy.

   Ideally, men should consume 420 mg. daily; women need only 320 mg. Eat some of these foods to maintain adequate magnesium levels:

   a. Leafy green vegetables

   b. Pumpkin seeds

   c. Avocados

   d. Almonds

   e. High-fat yogurts

2. *Sodium*: The amount of sodium required differs from other diet plans because other plans generally focus on less sodium. The sodium is lost with the water loss, so you will need to increase the sodium intake to keep the right balance of electrolytes. This is crucial especially during the initial phase of the diet. Gain sodium in these ways:

   a. Drinking bone broth regularly

   b. Adding salt to your food - Himalayan sea salt is a good choice.

   c. Enjoy more sodium-rich foods including eggs and red meats

   Be sure to monitor your blood pressure because the sodium can have an effect on your pressure if you're are prone to hypertension.

3. *Potassium*: Your normal blood pressure, regular heart rate, and fluid balance are aided by potassium. You need to remain cautious about adding potassium supplements to your diet because too much can cause an overload which could be toxic. Eat the following foods instead:

   a. Salmon

b. Mushrooms

c. Avocados

d. Leafy greens

e. Nuts

4. *Calcium*: Strong bones, muscle contraction, and proper blood clotting are all elements involved with calcium. Use these sources to add to your calcium counts:

a. Leafy greens such as broccoli

b. Dairy & non-dairy milk – unsweetened & zero carbs

You may need to supplement with calcium supplements including Vitamin D which is necessary for absorption. Both women and men should consume approximately 1000 mg. daily of calcium.

Vitamin D: Nutrients and hormones in your body are supplied by Vitamin D. You cannot always get enough from your food, but you can go outside and take in some healthy sunshine for your portion. Use caution from over-exposure and the risks of skin cancer. The vitamin D also helps your body to absorb magnesium, calcium and other essential minerals to maintain your muscle growth and bone density. If yours' is low; you are similar to about 1/3 of all Americans.

Supplement by adding 400 IU per day as recommended and add some fatty fish and mushrooms to your diet plan.

Fish Oil: Purchase this at any health food store in either the liquid or capsule form. The oil provides a natural anti-inflammatory content and also contributes to the higher fat intake requirements on the ketogenic diet.

MCT Oils and Ketosis: Medium chain triglycerides – more commonly known as MCT oils - are unique fatty acids found in its natural form in palm and coconut oil. Its advantages include:

- The oil helps lower your blood sugar.
- The use of MCTs makes it much easier to get into – and remain in ketosis.
- It's a natural anti-convulsive.
- It is also excellent for appetite control and weight loss.

Acetyl L-Carnitine: The carnitine helps muscle cells drive energy efficiently from fat metabolism because a lower level of the carnitine causes a reduced ability to use fat for energy. You need to keep the levels up to remain in ketosis.

CoQ10: Coenzyme Q10 is the technical term for this powerful antioxidant. It is also central molecule in your cellular process of creating energy. You can supplement your diet with 100 to 300 mg each day.

Creatine: This amino acid is favored by bodybuilders and athletes. It can be purchased either from a health food store or online with Amazon. Its most beneficial feature is for strengthening and building lean muscle mass as well as enhancing athletic performance.

Glutamine: Eight grams daily — taken orally — immediately after your workout — can help promote the production of glucose during exercise. When you purchase glutamine, don't purchase the powders because they usually have additives or sugar content.

Greens/Veggie Supplements: The best way to get the greens in your keto diet is through meals such as spinach in your eggs or a low-carb veggie juice with a cheese snack. Have a salad with dinner. However, if you don't like greens; you can purchase a greens supplement. A measured scoop of a protein shake will help with the issue.

Perfect Keto: You can use this powdered drink supplement to help spike your ketone levels. Don't be mistaken; this cannot replace the keto diet plan. It is a good stand-by if you exceed your carb limit. It can only assist to keep you in ketosis.

Vanadium and Chromium: Chromium and Vanadium are both trace minerals which are essential to the production of insulin which will stabilize your body's blood sugar level.

Whole Foods for Keto Supplements

Apple Cider Vinegar (ACV): A typical carbohydrate meal can be reduced by 31% with the use of this acetic acid by reducing the glycemic response. ACV also contains enzymes that will enhance the metabolism of fats and proteins.

You can add it full-strength or use an 8-ounce glass of water with 1 to 2 tablespoons of vinegar. These are some of the ways you can benefit from consuming ACV:

- Improves digestion

- Strengthens your immune system

- Great for detoxification

- Reduces cholesterol

- Good energy booster

- Helps you lose weight

- Helps relieve sore muscles

- Aids in diabetes/controls blood sugar

- Balances your inner body system

Bone Broth: This treat has been around for many years. The broth can eliminate keto flu symptoms and provide you with an increase of your essential electrolytes. These are just several of the benefits:

a. Boosting your immune system

b. Keeping your intestinal tract healthier

c. Increases collagen levels to improve your eyes, heart, skin, joints, and bone. You will also achieve improved brain health.

Make you a batch anytime to sip or use in your cooking. Use the recipe below:

Yields: 6-8 cups

Prep & Cooking Time: 6 hours – 45 minutes

Nutritional Facts Per Cup: Calories: 72 | Fat: 6 g | Net Carbs: 0.7 g | Protein: 3.6 g

What You Need

3 ½ lb. mixed assorted bones – ex. marrow bones, chicken feet or your choice

1 tbsp. pink Himalayan salt

1 med. of each:

-Parsnip

-White onion – skin on

5 peeled garlic cloves

2 med. of each:

-Celery stalks

-Carrots

2 tbsp. apple cider vinegar or lemon juice

8 c. of water

How to Prepare

1. Peel and slice the vegetables with roots into 1/3-inch pieces. Slice the onion in half. Chop the celery into thirds. Add the bay leaves into the slow cooker.

2. Toss in the chosen bones (can also be pork). Pour the water up to ¾ capacity – along with the juice/vinegar, and bay leaves. Sprinkle with the salt.

3. Secure the lid. Choose either low (ten hours) or high (six hours). You can simmer up to 48 hours.

4. Use a strainer to remove the bits of veggies. Set the bones aside to chill. Shred the meat and use as desired.

5. Refrigerate the broth overnight. Scrape away the tallow (greasy layer) if desired. Use within five days or freeze. You can also keep it in the canning jars for up to 45 days.

Probiotics: You can eat kimchee, Greek yogurt, kefir or similar fermented foods. You can also take a supplement.

Fermented Foods: Foods such as coconut water kefir or coconut milk kefir, pickles, sauerkraut, and kimchee are beneficial to your digestive system. The natural acids also help stabilize your blood sugar levels as well as the enzymes, probiotics, and other bioactive nutrients help support ketosis. These are three excellent reasons you should consume fermented foods. Fermented foods help restore the 'good' bacteria in your gut.

Lemon and Lime: These are two citric acid filled supplements to consider to reduce your blood sugar levels naturally. The trace minerals in lemon and lime, such as potassium, are present to improve your insulin — signaling a boost in your liver function.

You can use them in many ways including overcooked veggies or meats, in your green juices, or with your salad to improve your state of ketosis.

- Boosts your immune system
- Blood purifier
- Balances pH
- Reduces fever
- Flushes out unwanted materials
- Excellent for weight loss
- Decreases blemishes and wrinkles

- Relieves respiratory infections
- Reduces toothache pain

Chlorella: The green algae superfood is good for fighting off fatigue. It contains Chlorella Growth Factor – a nutrient containing DNA and RNA to help increase energy transport between your cells. You can purchase the supplement in powder form, tablets, or capsules. Mix it with water, a smoothie, or other drinks and have one daily.

Spirulina: The blue-green algae is similar to chlorella and contains all the amino acids your body requires which makes it a complete protein. It also contains magnesium, iron, potassium and other beneficial nutrients. It has superb antioxidant properties. The medication has shown positive results with individuals who suffer from cholesterol and high blood pressure. It will raise the HDL (good cholesterol) and lower the LDL (bad cholesterol). You can purchase in capsule form or in powder to mix in water or with a tasty smoothie.

Turmeric: The use or this Asian orange herb dates back to Ayurveda and Chinese medicine. The curcumin (an anti-inflammatory compound) found in the turmeric helps improve your insulin receptor function while regulating your blood sugar levels. Add turmeric to your meats, vegetables, green drinks, or smoothies. To maximize the antioxidant elements, add the turmeric after the meal is finished cooking.

Turmeric has many health benefits:

- Reduces the cholesterol level
- Weight management
- Prevents Alzheimer's disease
- Relieves arthritis
- Controls diabetes
- Improves digestion

The Not-So-Often Foods

You may use these occasionally, but you need to realize they can add extra carbs to your recipes. To name a few of the forbidden 'some-timers;' here they are:

- Beans and Legumes: This group to avoid includes peas, lentils, kidney beans, and chickpeas. If you use them; be sure to count the carbs, protein, and fat content.

- Agave Nectar: One teaspoon has 5 grams of carbs versus 4 grams of table sugar.

- Nut or Seed-Based Products: These items should be monitored since they contain high inflammatory Omega-6s which include corn oil, sunflower oil, almonds, pine nuts or walnuts.

- Cashews and Pistachios: The high carb content should be monitored for these yummy nuts.

- Hydrogenated Fats: Cold-pressed items should be avoided when using vegetable oils such as safflower, olive, soybean, or flax. Coronary heart disease has been linked to these fats which also include margarine.

- Potatoes and potato products

- Corn and corn products

- Fruits: Raspberries, blueberries, and cranberries contain a high sugar content. In small portions; you can enjoy some strawberries, apples, or pears.

- Alcohol Beverages: Limit the intake of your alcoholic drinks to include:

  a. Cocktails

  b. Flavored liquor

    c. Beer

    d. Dry Wine

    e. Mixers: Soda, Juice, or Syrup

- Diet Soda: Artificial sweeteners can cause you to go out of ketosis if you consume large amounts of diet drinks. Therefore, you have to use moderation. Research has shown a link between artificial sweeteners and sugar cravings, making it more challenging to curb those types of drink.

You should also avoid sugar including these:

- Dextrose
- Corn syrup
- Fructose
- Honey Maltose
- Maple syrup

On the other side of the issue, some professionals believe these spirits are acceptable:

- Whiskey, corn, barley, rye, and wheat are the grains used which have zero carbs or sugar.

- Rum: Choose the ones with zero carbs or sugar.

- Vodka: Check the carb content since it is usually produced (grain-based) from potatoes, rye, and wheat.

- Tequila: The agave plant is the source of tequila.

Note: The alcohol listing doesn't promote you drinking alcohol, but alcohol does produce ketones in the liver. Remember, it still needs to be consumed in small amounts to prevent any health issues.

Chapter 5:

Keto Breakfast Goodies

Blueberry Pancakes

Yields: 5 Servings

Nutritional Facts: 311.4 Cal. | 15.25 g Protein | 22.61 g Fat | 5.78 g Net Carbs

What You Need

½ t. vanilla extract

¾ c. ricotta

¼ t. salt

3 large eggs

¼ c. unsweetened vanilla almond milk

1 t. baking powder

1 c. almond flour

¼ - ½ t. stevia powder

½ c. golden flaxseed meal

¼ c. blueberries

How to Prepare

1. Warm up a skillet using the medium heat setting. Combine the ricotta, eggs, milk, and vanilla extract. Blend the stevia, baking powder, flour, salt, and flaxseed meal in another dish.

2. Add the dry with the wet ingredients into a blender, slowly, until a batter forms. For each ¼ cup of batter; add two to three blueberries.

3. Add butter to the skillet. When it melts, pour the batter in and brown. Flip when browned. Serve with additional berries or a drizzle of sugar-free syrup.

Crispy Light Waffles – Grain-Free

Yields: 8 Servings

Nutritional Facts: 140.0 Cal. | 4.0 g Prot. | 11.0 g Fat | 1.0 g Net Carbs

What You Need

2/3 c. almond flour

1 t. xanthan gum

¼ c. coconut flour

1 tbsp. psyllium husk

1 c. water

¼ c. coconut oil/butter

3 tbsp. xylitol/swerve

¼ t. kosher salt

3 eggs

1 t. vanilla extract

1 ½ t. baking powder

Suggestions for Serving Ingredients

Sugar-free syrup

Butter

Berries

Also Needed: Waffle Iron

How to Prepare

1. In a medium mixing container – add the coconut flour, almond flour, xanthan gum, and psyllium husk. Set aside for now.

2. In a Dutch oven, warm up the water, sweetener, butter, and salt until it simmers. Reduce the heat and whisk in the flour mixture. Stir until it forms a ball (1-3 min.).

3. Arrange the dough in the bowl to cool five minutes. You want the dough to be warm, not hot.

4. Lightly beat the eggs and add one egg at a time. Blend with an electric mixer. Stir in the baking powder, and vanilla extract. It should form an elastic-type dough. Let the dough rest about ten minutes.

5. Warm up the waffle iron using the high-temperature setting.

6. Grease the iron and spoon in the batter. Close the iron (8-12 min.) until golden.

7. The dough is good for a day or two in the fridge. The waffles are good for three days at room temperature.

Eggs Benedict & Bacon

Yields: 2 Servings

Nutritional Facts: 585 Calories | 19 g Protein | 54 g Fat | 1.5 Net Carbs

What You Need for the Mug Cake

1 large egg

2 tbsp. butter

½ t. baking powder

3 tbsp. almond flour

¼ t. of each:

      -Onion powder

      -Chili powder

To Taste: Pepper & salt

What You Need for the Topping

3 large eggs

4 bacon slices

2 tbsp. hollandaise sauce

Dash of salt & pepper

How to Prepare

1. Combine all of the cake fixings into a round dish or mug. Microwave for 1 ½ minutes or until done and puffed. Tap the mug/cup gently – upside down to remove the cake. Slice in half and set aside.

2. Prepare the bacon until thoroughly over the med-high stovetop setting. Poach two eggs.

3. Assemble by adding two bacon slices and one poached egg on half of the mug cake. Add one tablespoon of hollandaise sauce and enjoy

French Toast & Keto Almond Bread

Yields: 4 Servings

Nutritional Facts: 348 Cal. | 33 g Fat| 11 g Protein| 2 g Net Carbs

What You Need for the French Toast

2 medium whisked eggs

4 slices bread (full recipe below)

1 tbsp. coconut milk/water

Dash of cinnamon & nutmeg

Stevia to taste

For Cooking: 2 tbsp ghee/coconut oil

How to Prepare

1. Combine the water, eggs, stevia, cinnamon, and nutmeg. Dip each slice of bread into the mixture.

2. Prepare a frying pan with the coconut oil and add two slices of bread to the pan. Cook about 40 seconds and flip for another 40 seconds. Continue until the second batch is done.

3. Serve with some berries or ghee.

Keto Almond Bread for French Toast

Yields: 4 Servings

Nutritional Facts: 257 Cal. | 24 g Fat | 8 g Protein | 2 g Net Carbs

What You Need

1 c. almond flour

2 whisked eggs

1 ½ t. baking powder

3 tbsp. olive oil

Also Needed: 3.5x8-in. baking tin

How to Prepare

1. Program the oven temperature to 350ºF. Grease the baking pan.

2. Combine all of the fixings to form a sticky dough. Arrange into the greased tin and bake 30 minutes.

3. Carefully, 'tip-out' the bread and slice into four squares – similar to flatbread.

Pumpkin Maple Flaxseed Muffins

Yields: 10 Servings

Nutritional Facts: 120.0 Cal. | 8.5 g Fat | 5.0 g Protein | 2.0 g Net Carbs

What You Need

1 ¼ c. ground flaxseeds

½ tbsp. baking powder

1/3 c. erythritol

1 tbsp. of each:

> -Cinnamon

> -Pumpkin pie spice

½ t. salt

2 tbsp. coconut oil

1 c. pure pumpkin puree

1 egg

½ t. of each:

> -Vanilla extract

> -Apple cider vinegar

¼ c. maple syrup

Also Needed:

-Blender such as NutriBullet

-Muffin tin – 10 sections with silicone liners

Garnish: Pumpkin seeds

How to Prepare

1. Program the oven temperature to 350°F. Prepare the muffin tin with cupcake liners.

2. Add the seeds to the blender about one second – no longer or it could become damp. Combine the dry fixings and whisk until well mixed.

3. Add the puree, vanilla extract, and pumpkin spice along with the maple syrup (½ t.) if using. Blend in the oil, egg, and apple cider vinegar. Combine nuts or any other fold-ins of your choice, but also add the carbs.

4. Scoop the mixture out by the tablespoon into the prepared tins. Garnish with some of the pumpkin seeds. Leave a little space in the top since they will rise. Bake approximately 20 minutes.

5. They are ready when they are slightly browned. Let them cool a few minutes and add some ghee/butter or some more syrup.

Chapter 6:

Lunchtime Favorites

Caprese Salad

Yields: 4 Servings

Nutritional Facts: Cal: 190.75 |4.58 g Net Carbs| 7.71 g Protein| 63.49 g Fat

What You Need

3 c. grape tomatoes

4 peeled garlic cloves

2 tbsp. avocado oil

10 pearl-sized mozzarella balls

4 c. baby spinach leaves

¼ c. fresh basil leaves

1 tbsp. of each:

   -Brine reserved from the cheese

-Pesto

How to Prepare

1. Use some aluminum foil to cover a baking tray. Program the oven to 400°F. Arrange the cloves and tomatoes on the baking pan and drizzle with the oil. Bake 20-30 minutes until the tops are slightly browned.

2. Drain the liquid (saving one tablespoon) from the mozzarella. Mix the pesto with the brine.

3. Arrange the spinach in a large serving bowl. Transfer the tomatoes to the dish along with the roasted garlic. Drizzle with the pesto sauce.

4. Garnish with the mozzarella balls, and freshly torn basil leaves.

Egg Drop Soup

Yields: 6 Servings

Nutritional Facts: 255 Cal. | 2.9 g Net Carbs | 22.4 g Fat | 10.8 g Protein

What You Need

2 quarts vegetable broth

1 tbsp. freshly grated each:

-Ginger

-Turmeric

1 small sliced chili pepper

2 tbsp. coconut aminos

2 minced garlic cloves

4 large eggs

2 c. sliced mushrooms

4 c. chopped spinach/swiss chard

2 med. sliced spring onions

6 tbsp. EVOO

2 tbsp. freshly chopped cilantro

Black pepper to taste

1 t. salt ex. Pink Himalayan

How to Prepare

1. Mince the garlic cloves and slice the peppers and mushrooms. Grate the ginger root and turmeric.

2. Chop the chard stalks and leaves. Separate the stalks from the leaves. Dump the vegetable stock into a soup pot and simmer until it begins to boil. Toss in the garlic, ginger, turmeric, chard stalks, mushrooms, coconut aminos, and chili peppers. Boil for around five minutes.

3. Fold in the chard leaves and simmer for one minute.

4. Whip the eggs in a dish and add them slowly to the soup mixture. Stir until the egg is done and set it on the counter.

5. Slice the onions and chop the cilantro. Toss them into the pot.

6. Pour into serving bowls and drizzle with some olive oil (1 tbsp. for each serving).

7. Serve warm or chilled, and store in a closed bowl for up to five days.

Lemon Garlic Shrimp Pasta

Yields: 4 Servings

Nutritional Facts: 360 Cal. | 3.5 g Net Carbs | 21 g Fat | 36 g Protein

What You Need

2 bags angel hair pasta

4 garlic cloves

2 tbsp. each:

   -Olive oil

   -Butter

½ lemon

1 lb. large raw shrimp

½ t. paprika

Fresh basil

Pepper and salt

How to Prepare

1. Drain the water from the package of noodles and rinse them in cold water. Add them to a pot of boiling water for two minutes. Transfer them to a hot skillet over medium heat to remove the excess liquid (dry roast). Set them to the side.

2. Use the same pan to warm the oil, butter, and smashed garlic. Sauté a few minutes but don't brown.

3. Slice the lemon into rounds and add them to the garlic along with the shrimp. Sauté for approximately three minutes per side.

4. Add the noodles and spices and stir to blend the flavors.

Sushi

Yields: 3 Servings

Cal: 353 | Protein: 18.3 g | Net Carbs: 5.7 g | Fat: 25.7 g

What You Need

5 oz. smoked salmon/any seafood

16 oz. cauliflower

1 tbsp. coconut Aminos

1 cucumber (6 in.)

1 pkg. cream cheese – softened (6 oz.)

1 to 2 tbsp. unseasoned rice vinegar

5 Nori sheets

½ med avocado

Also Needed:

-Food processor

-Bamboo roller

How to Prepare

1. Pulse the cauliflower into rice-sized bits.

2. Cut up the cucumber first – end to end. Hold it upright and slice off each side. Trash the middle piece (or use it in a salad). Also, slice two side pieces into strips. Put in the refrigerator.

3. Prepare a hot pan and cook the cauliflower rice. Sprinkle with approximately one tablespoon of the aminos.

4. When done, add the rice to a bowl with the cream cheese and vinegar. Stir well and place in the fridge.

5. Slice one-half of the avocado into strips. Scoop the shell.

6. Place a nori sheet on a bamboo roller covered with saran wrap. Spread the mixture on the nori sheet, add the fillings, and roll. Be sure it's tight.

Thai Pork Salad

Yields: 2 Servings

Nutritional Facts: 461 Cal. | 5.2 g Net Carbs | 32.6 g Fat | 29.2 g Protein

What You Need for the Salad

2 c. romaine lettuce

10 oz. pulled pork

¼ medium chopped red bell pepper

¼ c. chopped cilantro

What You Need for the Sauce

2 tbsp. of each:

-Tomato paste

-Chopped cilantro

Juice & zest of 1 lime

2 tbsp. (+) 2 t. soy sauce

1 t. of each:

-Red curry paste

-Five Spice

-Fish sauce

¼ t. red pepper flakes

1 tbsp. (+) 1 t. rice wine vinegar

½ t. mango extract

10 drops liquid stevia

How to Prepare

1. Zest half of the lime and chop the cilantro.
2. Mix all of the sauce fixings.

3. Blend the barbecue sauce components and set aside.

4. Pull the pork apart and make the salad. Pour a glaze over the pork with a bit of the sauce.

Chapter 7:

Dinnertime Specialties

BBQ Pulled Beef Sando in the Slow Cooker

Yields: 4 Servings

Nutritional Facts: 184 Cal. | 3.6 g Net Carbs | 15.1 g Fat | 5.1 g Protein

What You Need

3 lbs. boneless chuck roast

2 t. of each:

     -Garlic powder

     -Pink Himalayan salt

1 t. of each:

     -Black pepper

     -Onion powder

1 tbsp. smoked paprika

¼ c. apple cider vinegar

2 tbsp. of each:

-Tomato paste

-Coconut Aminos

½ c. bone broth – see below

¼ c. melted butter

How to Prepare

1. Remove all of the fat from the beef and cut it half to fit in the cooker.

2. Combine the pepper, salt, and paprika along with the garlic and onion powder. Rub the beef and arrange the pieces in the pot.

3. In another container, melt the butter and whisk in the Aminos, vinegar, and tomato paste. Pour the mixture over the roast and add the bone broth.

4. Set on the low setting to cook for 10-12 hours.

5. Once it's done, increase the temperature setting to high and let the sauce thicken. Shred the beef and add it back and toss. Enjoy!

Bone Broth for the BBQ in the Slow Cooker

Broth Servings: 8

Nutrients included in the BBQ recipe above

What You Need

Purified water

1 tbsp. vinegar – white or apple cider

Bones from grass-fed beef

How to Prepare

1. Add all of the bones to a large slow cooker, and cover with the water.

2. Pour in the vinegar.

3. Set the pot on the low setting for six hours (minimum).

4. *Note:* Beef can simmer 48 hours or chicken 24 hours.

5. Empty the broth through a sieve into a container. Remove the bones with a pair of tongs.

6. Add some salt and pepper to taste. You can use it for up to one week or freeze for another recipe later.

Cheeseburger Calzone

Yields: 8 Servings

Nutritional Facts: 580 Cal. | 3.0 g Carbs | 34.0 g Protein | 47.0 g Fat

What You Need

½ yellow diced onion

1 ½ lb. ground beef – lean

4 thick-cut bacon strips

4 dill pickle spears

8 oz. cream cheese – divided

1 egg

½ c. mayonnaise

1 c. of each:

-Shredded cheddar cheese

-Almond flour

-Shredded mozzarella cheese

How to Prepare

1. Program the oven to 425°F. Prepare a cookie tin with parchment paper.

2. Chop the pickles into spears. Set aside for now.

3. Prepare the crust. Combine ½ of the cream cheese and the mozzarella cheese. Microwave 35 seconds. When it melts, add the egg and almond flour to make the dough. Set aside.

4. Cook the beef on the stove using medium heat.

5. Cook the bacon (microwave for five minutes or stovetop). When cool, break into bits.

6. Dice the onion and add to the beef and cook until softened. Toss in the bacon, cheddar cheese, pickle bits, the rest of the cream cheese, and mayonnaise. Stir well.

7. Roll the dough onto the prepared baking tin. Scoop the mixture into the center. Fold the ends and side to make the calzone.

8. Bake until browned or about 15 minutes. Let it rest for 10 minutes before slicing.

Fettuccine Chicken Alfredo

Yields: 2 Servings

Nutritional Facts: 585 Cal. | 1 g Net Carbs | 51 g Fat | 25 g Protein

What You Need

2 tbsp. butter

2 minced garlic cloves

½ t. dried basil

½ c. heavy cream

4 tbsp. grated parmesan

What You Need for the Chicken and Noodles

2 chicken thighs - no bones or skin

1 tbsp. olive oil

1 bag Miracle Noodle - Fettuccini

Salt and pepper

How to Prepare

1. For the Sauce: Add the cloves to a pan with the butter for two minutes. Empty the cream into the skillet and let it simmer two additional minutes. Toss in one tablespoon of the parmesan at a time. Add the pepper, salt, and dried basil. Simmer three to five minutes on the low heat setting.

2. For the Chicken: Pound the chicken with a meat tenderizer hammer until it is ½-inch thick. Warm up the oil in a skillet using the medium heat setting and put the chicken in to cook for about seven minutes per side. Shred and set aside.

3. For the Noodles: Prepare the package of noodles. Rinse, and boil them for two minutes in a pot of water.

4. Fold in the noodles along with the sauce and shredded chicken. Cook slowly for two minutes and enjoy.

Nacho Chicken Casserole

Yields: 6 Servings

Nutritional Facts: 426 Cal. | 32.2 g Fat | 4.3 g Net Carbs | 30.8 g Protein

What You Need

1 med. jalapeno pepper

1 ¾ lbs. chicken thighs

To Taste: Pepper and salt

2 tbsp. olive oil

1 ½ t. chili seasoning

4 oz. of each:

>   -Cheddar cheese

>   -Cream cheese

3 tbsp. parmesan cheese

1 c. green chilies and tomatoes

¼ c. sour cream

1 pkg. frozen cauliflower

Also Needed: Immersion blender

How to Prepare

1. Warm up the oven to 375°F.
2. Slice the jalapeno into bits and set aside.
3. Remove the skin and bones from the chicken. Chop it up and add some pepper and salt. Cook in olive oil on med-high until browned.
4. Blend in the sour cream, cream cheese, and ¾ of the cheddar cheese. Stir until melted and combined well. Pour in the tomatoes and chilies. Stir and add it all to a baking dish.
5. Cook the cauliflower in the microwave until done. Blend in the rest of the cheese with the immersion blender until it resembles mashed potatoes. Season as desired.
6. Spread the cauliflower concoction over the casserole and sprinkle with the peppers. Bake approximately 15-20 minutes.

Stuffed Pork Chops

Yields: 4 Servings

Nutritional Facts: 778 Cal. | 1 g Net Carbs | 102 g Protein | 38 g Fat

What You Need

3 slices bacon

4 thick cut pork chops

3 oz. of each:

-Feta cheese

-Bleu cheese

2 oz. cream cheese

1/3 c. green onion

To Taste:

-Salt

-Garlic powder

-Black pepper

How to Prepare

1. Program the oven temperature to 350°F. Lightly grease a baking tin.

2. Cook the bacon, reserve the grease and set aside.

3. Mix the feta and bleu cheese. Blend in the onions and bacon. Next, add the cream cheese, and mix well.

4. Split the non-fat side of the pork and add the cheese mixture – closing with a toothpick. Sprinkle with the garlic powder, salt, and pepper.

5. Sear with the bacon grease in the skillet for 1-½ minutes per side.

6. Arrange the chops on the baking pan and cook for 55 minutes.

7. Let the chops rest about three minutes.

Chapter 8:

On-the-Go

If you live a hectic lifestyle as many individuals and families do in today's fast-paced society; some of these choices will help you along the way:

Eating-Out Strategies

Going out to eat is fun but be smart and do some online research before you leave the house. Many of the restaurants now have an online presence to make dieting a less scary adventure. As you continue with your pre-planning, it will become easier, and you can branch out to other locations with the knowledge gained.

These are a few recommendations that might help:

Breakfast: Sometimes, there is nothing better than eggs if you want to play it safe. You may be off on some of the counts but after you have used some of the recipes in this book; you will know how to gauge your eating habits for the most important meal of the day.

Lunch: Chicken and fish are usually good choices. Many of the restaurants now offer diet-friendly menus. Select a chicken salad or a regular salad. Just be cautious of the dressing used. Try some vinaigrette or plain vinegar.

Dinner: Always choose a fresh green veggie with a lean cut of meat as your main course. Try something in the line of a hamburger minus the bun, or a tempting entrée of broccoli and steak. Tasty!

A Word of Caution: Wheat products contain an enormous amount of carbs. This will eliminate a pita or a tortilla, baked potato, or a plate of French fries. Ask for a substitute with another side dish. Most restaurants will be happy to accommodate your request, especially if he/she knows you are on a special diet plan.

Know How to Control the Cravings

Essentially, your body is saying it needs a nutrient when you have a particular craving. Leave the carb-enriched treats behind and find a new path. Keep these ideas in mind:

What You are Craving	Your Body Needs	Eat This
Carbs, Bread, Pasta	Nitrogen	High Protein Meat

Chocolate	Magnesium Carbon Chromium	Nuts & Seeds Spinach Broccoli & Cheese
Salty Foods	Silicon	Nuts & Cheese
Oil & Fatty Foods	Chloride Calcium	Fish Broccoli, Spinach, & Cheese
Sugary Foods	Tryptophan Phosphorus Sulfur	Liver, Cheese, Lamb Eggs, Beef, Chicken Broccoli, Cauliflower

Travel Tips

Traveling and depending on other people to cook for you can sometimes pose an issue. These are some suggestions that might apply to your situation:

Carbs: Stay away from bread, pasta, and baked goods. They will be tempting if you are away from home. If you slip and have a tasty treat that isn't in your plan, just test with a Ketostix kit (available at Walmart) and get back in gear.

MCT Oil: Use one or two servings of the oil in your tea or similar drink prior to noon to keep your beta hydroxyl butyrate high. This is what will retain you in ketosis.

Now it is time to open the door to your new lifestyle plan using your ketogenic diet plan!

Conclusion

Thanks for reading your entire copy of the book, *Ketogenic Diet for Beginners and Keto Lifestyle Plan: All You Need to Know to Control Weight and to Live A Healthy Life.* Let's hope, as you read through your personal copy, that it was informative and provided you with all of the tools you need to achieve your goals of controlling your weight and enjoying a healthier lifestyle.

The next step is to recall the essential foods along with the 'not so good' items on the ketogenic diet plan. Compile a shopping list of all of the items you want to prepare for a couple of days. All of the nutritional counts are provided within each of the recipes, so just stay within the carbohydrate limitations of your chosen type of plan.

Remain strong-minded and stick to your goals during your transition to ketosis. Each of the recipes in this diet plan has been researched with your goals in mind. Follow the directions and recipe preparation methods. Before long, you will be exercising and cooking much healthier meals for you and your family. Set your goals and know how your body will react to the changes it will make during the process.

You are human and sometimes will slip with a hot fudge sundae or a piece of strawberry shortcake. If you do, just get back on the right path and let it go. Life happens; you might just need a little longer to get the diet into motion while you lose those cravings. You will be too full to worry about consuming the wasted calories for one simple treat. Move forward; tomorrow is a fresh day.

After you have started losing your weight, it's important to have a bit of fun. However, you should be sure it is not a food-related treat unless it's keto-friendly. Buy a new outfit to show off your weight loss. Take the family for an evening on the town. You deserve it.

Finally, if you found this book useful in any way, a review on Amazon is always appreciated!

Index for the Recipes

2. Cheeseburger Calzone

3. Fettuccine Chicken Alfredo

4. Nacho Chicken Casserole

5. Stuffed Pork Chops

Description

Have you tried other diet plans to discover that you were always hungry? It is great to know that you're all geared up and ready to start losing weight and changing over to a healthier way of preparing your foods. If you have tried the rest, maybe it is time to use the Ketogenic Diet Plan that everyone is buzzing about. It really does work!

The *Ketogenic Diet for Beginners and Keto Lifestyle Plan: All You Need to Know to Control Weight and to Live A Healthy Life* has a selection of recipes for breakfast, lunch, and dinner. Each recipe has a detailed step-by-step process described providing you with the calories, protein, net carbs, and fats. It's never been easier to serve healthy meals and enjoy the benefits provided by the keto diet plan.

You will also learn how the plan works and how to balance an exercise plan with your eating habits. A list is provided of a few supplements and foods you can eat to keep your body in ketosis.

Be the envy of the neighbors and throw a party to show off your new way of eating today and enjoy your new *Ketogenic Diet Plan*. Here is a sneak peak of what you are missing if you don't add this book to your library:

- Eggs Benedict & Bacon
- Fettuccine Chicken Alfredo
- Nacho Chicken Casserole
- French Toast & Keto Almond Bread

With determination, you will soon reach your goals! All you need to do is add this valuable collection to your personal library to enjoy anytime.

Made in the USA
Columbia, SC
20 May 2018